Brave Leadership Mastery Journal

Tony Bodoh

Published by Tony Bodoh International, LLC

Contact the publisher at www.TonyBodoh.com.

Disclaimer: This publication and the content provided herein are simply for educational purposes, and do not take the place of legal advice from your attorney or the advice of a competent professional who knows your specific situation. Every effort has been made to ensure that the content provided in this book is accurate and helpful for our readers at publishing time. However, this is not an exhaustive treatment of the subjects. No liability is assumed for losses or damages due to the information provided. You are responsible for your own choices, actions, and results.

ISBN-13: 9781795802765

Dedication

This Brave Leadership Mastery Journal is dedicated to the person you are being right now and to the person you are becoming as you use this journal.

Always remember that in every moment, you have the power to make a decision. That power means every moment of your life contains within it the potential to alter the trajectory of human history.

You Can Be A Brave Leader

Here's what I know about you: Because you are reading this, you are a leader or you are interested in being a leader. I also know that you are facing some real challenges in your life or in business that require you to step outside your comfort zone. Maybe these challenges have even shaken you to your core. Based on my experience, I believe that you have to become a new and different person so you can achieve the goals you have set your heart and mind on.

I have been exactly where you are. That's why I created this journal and the body of work I call Brave Leadership Mastery™.

My journey in Brave Leadership Mastery started in 2008. I had job that I was really good at and paid well to do. I had a wonderful family with a wife and two little girls. I had a nice home and two cars.

On the outside everything looked great. But, what no one knew was that every morning when I went to work I felt like I had to check my soul at the door. I felt like I was called to head in one direction and the path I was on with the company I worked for was headed in another, very different, direction. My stress levels were so bad by that point that I developed allergies which were triggering anaphylaxis three to four times a week. Worse yet, my doctors had no answers for me.

That's when new circumstances arose.

It was the midst of the 2007-2009 financial crisis. The company I worked for offered me an option. I could take a promotion, which sounded like more of the same, or I could leave the company with a modest severance package.

I chose the latter and started my own business as a customer experience consultant.

The story is much longer and there were many peaks and valleys along the way. However, my intense ten-year focus on studying and understanding human experiences through the context of customer, employee, and leader experiences led me to a discovery.

Brave people don't believe they are brave.

I was shocked when I realized that. Again and again, I found that those who truly made a decision to do something brave did not see themselves as brave. First responders, our service men and women in the military, entrepreneurs and executives, doctors and researchers, and even parents, who had done some brave thing all had a similar response when asked why they did it:

"I was just doing my job."

"It was the right thing to do."

"Anyone would have done the same thing."

When I pressed them for more, I found that they really believed in what they were saying. That was my, "Aha!" moment.

I finally realized that there is a difference between feeling courageous and being brave.

Let me break it down.

Feeling courageous means very literally to feel the emotion of courage. We can summon courage for a moment or we can develop a habit of feeling courageous and acting upon that feeling. There is nothing wrong with this. Many noble and good deeds are done because people have summoned the courage to do them.

Yet, courage is different than bravery.

The person who acts because they feel courage knows that they felt the courage and they can usually point to the emotion as the catalyst that caused them to act.

Brave leaders are different.

Bravery is not an emotion. It is a character trait. It is an intrinsic part of the fiber of the person who is brave. In fact, it is so much a part of them that they cannot see it in themselves. It is just who they are. That is why they assume it was just part of their job or that anyone else would do it. It is their self-image that tells them this is who they are and what they do. This self-image informs their worldview.

You might be thinking, "Well, I am not brave and I hardly ever feel courage when I really could use it."

That's okay. I admit that I still struggle to summon the courage to act when I face new challenges. There are many more parts of my life where I am not brave than where I am brave.

You see, what I learned while on my journey is that we can learn to summon courage. Then, if we do this repeatedly and consistently, we can develop the habit of courage. Once we have the habit of courage in an area of our lives, we can continue to practice courageous actions until our self-image changes and we become brave.

The Brave Leadership Mastery programs I facilitate help leaders learn how to:

- summon courage;
- develop the habit of courage; and,
- eventually become brave leaders

It is a process. An essential part of that process is the use of The Brave Leadership Mastery Journal which you now have in your hands.

While the four morning and five evening exercises in this 90-day journal may seem simple, they are powerful. They may only take a few minutes when you wake up and before you go to sleep, but I promise you that they are life-changing.

This method has been used by grade schoolers, elite military operators, Olympians, professional athletes, executives, and entrepreneurs. It works when you work it. Start with it today and do it consistently for 90 days and you will see your life and your business change.

In closing, I want to share the perspective that has driven me for many years.

I believe that in every moment of human experience each one of us has the power to make a decision. This power to decide means that we have the potential in every moment to alter the trajectory of human history.

You can either see this power and the potential in each moment as a tremendous burden or a fantastic opportunity. What I know is this: If you choose to act upon it to make the future better than the past, you will need to summon courage, develop the habit of acting courageously, and eventually become a brave leader.

If you'd like more guidance in how to use this journal we have both free resources you can use and courses or workshops you can enroll in at www.TonyBodoh.com/BLM

DAY #1 Date: ______

Morning Preparation

My long-term ***vision*** is:

This morning I am ***grateful*** for... and it is meaningful because:

Today I ***intend*** to be:

Today I will ***focus*** my attention on these tasks which will help me achieve my vision:

Evening Review

Today I intentionally performed this act of ***kindness*** and I learned:

Today I had these ***successes*** and they were meaningful because:

Today I decide to ***improve*** myself in this way:

To improve, I will be aware of this ***trigger*** happening in the future:

I ***decide*** now that if a similar trigger situation arises in the future, I will do this:

DAY #2 Date: ______

Morning Preparation

My long-term ***vision*** is:

This morning I am ***grateful*** for... and it is meaningful because:

Today I ***intend*** to be:

Today I will ***focus*** my attention on these tasks which will help me achieve my vision:

Evening Review

Today I intentionally performed this act of ***kindness*** and I learned:

Today I had these ***successes*** and they were meaningful because:

Today I decide to ***improve*** myself in this way:

To improve, I will be aware of this ***trigger*** happening in the future:

I ***decide*** now that if a similar trigger situation arises in the future, I will do this:

Day #3 Date: ______

Morning Preparation

My long-term ***vision*** is:

This morning I am ***grateful*** for... and it is meaningful because:

Today I ***intend*** to be:

Today I will ***focus*** my attention on these tasks which will help me achieve my vision:

Evening Review

Today I intentionally performed this act of ***kindness*** and I learned:

Today I had these ***successes*** and they were meaningful because:

Today I decide to ***improve*** myself in this way:

To improve, I will be aware of this ***trigger*** happening in the future:

I ***decide*** now that if a similar trigger situation arises in the future, I will do this:

DAY #4 Date: ______

Morning Preparation

My long-term ***vision*** is:

This morning I am ***grateful*** for... and it is meaningful because:

Today I ***intend*** to be:

Today I will ***focus*** my attention on these tasks which will help me achieve my vision:

Evening Review

Today I intentionally performed this act of ***kindness*** and I learned:

Today I had these ***successes*** and they were meaningful because:

Today I decide to ***improve*** myself in this way:

To improve, I will be aware of this ***trigger*** happening in the future:

I ***decide*** now that if a similar trigger situation arises in the future, I will do this:

Day #5 Date: ______

Morning Preparation

My long-term ***vision*** is:

This morning I am ***grateful*** for... and it is meaningful because:

Today I ***intend*** to be:

Today I will ***focus*** my attention on these tasks which will help me achieve my vision:

Evening Review

Today I intentionally performed this act of ***kindness*** and I learned:

Today I had these ***successes*** and they were meaningful because:

Today I decide to ***improve*** myself in this way:

To improve, I will be aware of this ***trigger*** happening in the future:

I ***decide*** now that if a similar trigger situation arises in the future, I will do this:

DAY #6 Date: ______

Morning Preparation

My long-term ***vision*** is:

This morning I am ***grateful*** for... and it is meaningful because:

Today I ***intend*** to be:

Today I will ***focus*** my attention on these tasks which will help me achieve my vision:

Evening Review

Today I intentionally performed this act of ***kindness*** and I learned:

Today I had these ***successes*** and they were meaningful because:

Today I decide to ***improve*** myself in this way:

To improve, I will be aware of this ***trigger*** happening in the future:

I ***decide*** now that if a similar trigger situation arises in the future, I will do this:

DAY #7 Date: ______

Morning Preparation

My long-term ***vision*** is:

This morning I am ***grateful*** for... and it is meaningful because:

Today I ***intend*** to be:

Today I will ***focus*** my attention on these tasks which will help me achieve my vision:

Evening Review

Today I intentionally performed this act of ***kindness*** and I learned:

Today I had these ***successes*** and they were meaningful because:

Today I decide to ***improve*** myself in this way:

To improve, I will be aware of this ***trigger*** happening in the future:

I ***decide*** now that if a similar trigger situation arises in the future, I will do this:

DAY #8 Date: ______

Morning Preparation

My long-term ***vision*** is:

This morning I am ***grateful*** for... and it is meaningful because:

Today I ***intend*** to be:

Today I will ***focus*** my attention on these tasks which will help me achieve my vision:

Evening Review

Today I intentionally performed this act of ***kindness*** and I learned:

Today I had these ***successes*** and they were meaningful because:

Today I decide to ***improve*** myself in this way:

To improve, I will be aware of this ***trigger*** happening in the future:

I ***decide*** now that if a similar trigger situation arises in the future, I will do this:

DAY #9 Date: ______

Morning Preparation

My long-term ***vision*** is:

This morning I am ***grateful*** for... and it is meaningful because:

Today I ***intend*** to be:

Today I will ***focus*** my attention on these tasks which will help me achieve my vision:

Evening Review

Today I intentionally performed this act of ***kindness*** and I learned:

Today I had these ***successes*** and they were meaningful because:

Today I decide to ***improve*** myself in this way:

To improve, I will be aware of this ***trigger*** happening in the future:

I ***decide*** now that if a similar trigger situation arises in the future, I will do this:

DAY #10 Date: ______

Morning Preparation

My long-term ***vision*** is:

This morning I am ***grateful*** for... and it is meaningful because:

Today I ***intend*** to be:

Today I will ***focus*** my attention on these tasks which will help me achieve my vision:

Evening Review

Today I intentionally performed this act of ***kindness*** and I learned:

Today I had these ***successes*** and they were meaningful because:

Today I decide to ***improve*** myself in this way:

To improve, I will be aware of this ***trigger*** happening in the future:

I ***decide*** now that if a similar trigger situation arises in the future, I will do this:

DAY #11 Date: ______

Morning Preparation

My long-term ***vision*** is:

This morning I am ***grateful*** for... and it is meaningful because:

Today I ***intend*** to be:

Today I will ***focus*** my attention on these tasks which will help me achieve my vision:

Evening Review

Today I intentionally performed this act of ***kindness*** and I learned:

Today I had these ***successes*** and they were meaningful because:

Today I decide to ***improve*** myself in this way:

To improve, I will be aware of this ***trigger*** happening in the future:

I ***decide*** now that if a similar trigger situation arises in the future, I will do this:

DAY #12 Date: ______

Morning Preparation

My long-term ***vision*** is:

This morning I am ***grateful*** for... and it is meaningful because:

Today I ***intend*** to be:

Today I will ***focus*** my attention on these tasks which will help me achieve my vision:

Evening Review

Today I intentionally performed this act of ***kindness*** and I learned:

Today I had these ***successes*** and they were meaningful because:

Today I decide to ***improve*** myself in this way:

To improve, I will be aware of this ***trigger*** happening in the future:

I ***decide*** now that if a similar trigger situation arises in the future, I will do this:

DAY #13 Date: ______

Morning Preparation

My long-term ***vision*** is:

This morning I am ***grateful*** for... and it is meaningful because:

Today I ***intend*** to be:

Today I will ***focus*** my attention on these tasks which will help me achieve my vision:

Evening Review

Today I intentionally performed this act of ***kindness*** and I learned:

Today I had these ***successes*** and they were meaningful because:

Today I decide to ***improve*** myself in this way:

To improve, I will be aware of this ***trigger*** happening in the future:

I ***decide*** now that if a similar trigger situation arises in the future, I will do this:

DAY #14 Date: ______

Morning Preparation

My long-term ***vision*** is:

This morning I am ***grateful*** for... and it is meaningful because:

Today I ***intend*** to be:

Today I will ***focus*** my attention on these tasks which will help me achieve my vision:

Evening Review

Today I intentionally performed this act of ***kindness*** and I learned:

Today I had these ***successes*** and they were meaningful because:

Today I decide to ***improve*** myself in this way:

To improve, I will be aware of this ***trigger*** happening in the future:

I ***decide*** now that if a similar trigger situation arises in the future, I will do this:

DAY #15 Date: ______

Morning Preparation

My long-term ***vision*** is:

This morning I am ***grateful*** for... and it is meaningful because:

Today I ***intend*** to be:

Today I will ***focus*** my attention on these tasks which will help me achieve my vision:

Evening Review

Today I intentionally performed this act of ***kindness*** and I learned:

Today I had these ***successes*** and they were meaningful because:

Today I decide to ***improve*** myself in this way:

To improve, I will be aware of this ***trigger*** happening in the future:

I ***decide*** now that if a similar trigger situation arises in the future, I will do this:

DAY #16 Date: ______

Morning Preparation

My long-term ***vision*** is:

This morning I am ***grateful*** for... and it is meaningful because:

Today I ***intend*** to be:

Today I will ***focus*** my attention on these tasks which will help me achieve my vision:

Evening Review

Today I intentionally performed this act of ***kindness*** and I learned:

Today I had these ***successes*** and they were meaningful because:

Today I decide to ***improve*** myself in this way:

To improve, I will be aware of this ***trigger*** happening in the future:

I ***decide*** now that if a similar trigger situation arises in the future, I will do this:

Day #17 Date: ______

Morning Preparation

My long-term ***vision*** is:

This morning I am ***grateful*** for... and it is meaningful because:

Today I ***intend*** to be:

Today I will ***focus*** my attention on these tasks which will help me achieve my vision:

Evening Review

Today I intentionally performed this act of ***kindness*** and I learned:

Today I had these ***successes*** and they were meaningful because:

Today I decide to ***improve*** myself in this way:

To improve, I will be aware of this ***trigger*** happening in the future:

I ***decide*** now that if a similar trigger situation arises in the future, I will do this:

DAY #18 Date: ______

Morning Preparation

My long-term ***vision*** is:

This morning I am ***grateful*** for... and it is meaningful because:

Today I ***intend*** to be:

Today I will ***focus*** my attention on these tasks which will help me achieve my vision:

Evening Review

Today I intentionally performed this act of ***kindness*** and I learned:

Today I had these ***successes*** and they were meaningful because:

Today I decide to ***improve*** myself in this way:

To improve, I will be aware of this ***trigger*** happening in the future:

I ***decide*** now that if a similar trigger situation arises in the future, I will do this:

DAY #19 Date: ______

Morning Preparation

My long-term ***vision*** is:

This morning I am ***grateful*** for... and it is meaningful because:

Today I ***intend*** to be:

Today I will ***focus*** my attention on these tasks which will help me achieve my vision:

Evening Review

Today I intentionally performed this act of ***kindness*** and I learned:

Today I had these ***successes*** and they were meaningful because:

Today I decide to ***improve*** myself in this way:

To improve, I will be aware of this ***trigger*** happening in the future:

I ***decide*** now that if a similar trigger situation arises in the future, I will do this:

DAY #20 Date: ______

Morning Preparation

My long-term ***vision*** is:

This morning I am ***grateful*** for... and it is meaningful because:

Today I ***intend*** to be:

Today I will ***focus*** my attention on these tasks which will help me achieve my vision:

Evening Review

Today I intentionally performed this act of ***kindness*** and I learned:

Today I had these ***successes*** and they were meaningful because:

Today I decide to ***improve*** myself in this way:

To improve, I will be aware of this ***trigger*** happening in the future:

I ***decide*** now that if a similar trigger situation arises in the future, I will do this:

Day #21 Date: ______

Morning Preparation

My long-term ***vision*** is:

This morning I am ***grateful*** for... and it is meaningful because:

Today I ***intend*** to be:

Today I will ***focus*** my attention on these tasks which will help me achieve my vision:

Evening Review

Today I intentionally performed this act of ***kindness*** and I learned:

Today I had these ***successes*** and they were meaningful because:

Today I decide to ***improve*** myself in this way:

To improve, I will be aware of this ***trigger*** happening in the future:

I ***decide*** now that if a similar trigger situation arises in the future, I will do this:

Day #22 Date: ______

Morning Preparation

My long-term ***vision*** is:

This morning I am ***grateful*** for... and it is meaningful because:

Today I ***intend*** to be:

Today I will ***focus*** my attention on these tasks which will help me achieve my vision:

Evening Review

Today I intentionally performed this act of ***kindness*** and I learned:

Today I had these ***successes*** and they were meaningful because:

Today I decide to ***improve*** myself in this way:

To improve, I will be aware of this ***trigger*** happening in the future:

I ***decide*** now that if a similar trigger situation arises in the future, I will do this:

DAY #23 Date: ______

Morning Preparation

My long-term ***vision*** is:

This morning I am ***grateful*** for... and it is meaningful because:

Today I ***intend*** to be:

Today I will ***focus*** my attention on these tasks which will help me achieve my vision:

Evening Review

Today I intentionally performed this act of ***kindness*** and I learned:

Today I had these ***successes*** and they were meaningful because:

Today I decide to ***improve*** myself in this way:

To improve, I will be aware of this ***trigger*** happening in the future:

I ***decide*** now that if a similar trigger situation arises in the future, I will do this:

DAY #24 Date: ______

Morning Preparation

My long-term ***vision*** is:

This morning I am ***grateful*** for... and it is meaningful because:

Today I ***intend*** to be:

Today I will ***focus*** my attention on these tasks which will help me achieve my vision:

Evening Review

Today I intentionally performed this act of ***kindness*** and I learned:

Today I had these ***successes*** and they were meaningful because:

Today I decide to ***improve*** myself in this way:

To improve, I will be aware of this ***trigger*** happening in the future:

I ***decide*** now that if a similar trigger situation arises in the future, I will do this:

DAY #25 Date: ______

Morning Preparation

My long-term ***vision*** is:

This morning I am ***grateful*** for... and it is meaningful because:

Today I ***intend*** to be:

Today I will ***focus*** my attention on these tasks which will help me achieve my vision:

Evening Review

Today I intentionally performed this act of ***kindness*** and I learned:

Today I had these ***successes*** and they were meaningful because:

Today I decide to ***improve*** myself in this way:

To improve, I will be aware of this ***trigger*** happening in the future:

I ***decide*** now that if a similar trigger situation arises in the future, I will do this:

Day #26 Date: ______

Morning Preparation

My long-term ***vision*** is:

This morning I am ***grateful*** for... and it is meaningful because:

Today I ***intend*** to be:

Today I will ***focus*** my attention on these tasks which will help me achieve my vision:

Evening Review

Today I intentionally performed this act of ***kindness*** and I learned:

Today I had these ***successes*** and they were meaningful because:

Today I decide to ***improve*** myself in this way:

To improve, I will be aware of this ***trigger*** happening in the future:

I ***decide*** now that if a similar trigger situation arises in the future, I will do this:

DAY #27 Date: ______

Morning Preparation

My long-term ***vision*** is:

This morning I am ***grateful*** for... and it is meaningful because:

Today I ***intend*** to be:

Today I will ***focus*** my attention on these tasks which will help me achieve my vision:

Evening Review

Today I intentionally performed this act of ***kindness*** and I learned:

Today I had these ***successes*** and they were meaningful because:

Today I decide to ***improve*** myself in this way:

To improve, I will be aware of this ***trigger*** happening in the future:

I ***decide*** now that if a similar trigger situation arises in the future, I will do this:

DAY #28 Date: ______

Morning Preparation

My long-term ***vision*** is:

This morning I am ***grateful*** for... and it is meaningful because:

Today I ***intend*** to be:

Today I will ***focus*** my attention on these tasks which will help me achieve my vision:

Evening Review

Today I intentionally performed this act of ***kindness*** and I learned:

Today I had these ***successes*** and they were meaningful because:

Today I decide to ***improve*** myself in this way:

To improve, I will be aware of this ***trigger*** happening in the future:

I ***decide*** now that if a similar trigger situation arises in the future, I will do this:

DAY #29 Date: ______

Morning Preparation

My long-term ***vision*** is:

This morning I am ***grateful*** for... and it is meaningful because:

Today I ***intend*** to be:

Today I will ***focus*** my attention on these tasks which will help me achieve my vision:

Evening Review

Today I intentionally performed this act of ***kindness*** and I learned:

Today I had these ***successes*** and they were meaningful because:

Today I decide to ***improve*** myself in this way:

To improve, I will be aware of this ***trigger*** happening in the future:

I ***decide*** now that if a similar trigger situation arises in the future, I will do this:

DAY #30 Date: ______

Morning Preparation

My long-term ***vision*** is:

This morning I am ***grateful*** for... and it is meaningful because:

Today I ***intend*** to be:

Today I will ***focus*** my attention on these tasks which will help me achieve my vision:

Evening Review

Today I intentionally performed this act of ***kindness*** and I learned:

Today I had these ***successes*** and they were meaningful because:

Today I decide to ***improve*** myself in this way:

To improve, I will be aware of this ***trigger*** happening in the future:

I ***decide*** now that if a similar trigger situation arises in the future, I will do this:

DAY #31 Date: ______

Morning Preparation

My long-term ***vision*** is:

This morning I am ***grateful*** for... and it is meaningful because:

Today I ***intend*** to be:

Today I will ***focus*** my attention on these tasks which will help me achieve my vision:

Evening Review

Today I intentionally performed this act of ***kindness*** and I learned:

Today I had these ***successes*** and they were meaningful because:

Today I decide to ***improve*** myself in this way:

To improve, I will be aware of this ***trigger*** happening in the future:

I ***decide*** now that if a similar trigger situation arises in the future, I will do this:

Day #32 Date: ______

Morning Preparation

My long-term ***vision*** is:

This morning I am ***grateful*** for... and it is meaningful because:

Today I ***intend*** to be:

Today I will ***focus*** my attention on these tasks which will help me achieve my vision:

Evening Review

Today I intentionally performed this act of ***kindness*** and I learned:

Today I had these ***successes*** and they were meaningful because:

Today I decide to ***improve*** myself in this way:

To improve, I will be aware of this ***trigger*** happening in the future:

I ***decide*** now that if a similar trigger situation arises in the future, I will do this:

DAY #33 Date: ______

Morning Preparation

My long-term ***vision*** is:

This morning I am ***grateful*** for... and it is meaningful because:

Today I ***intend*** to be:

Today I will ***focus*** my attention on these tasks which will help me achieve my vision:

Evening Review

Today I intentionally performed this act of ***kindness*** and I learned:

Today I had these ***successes*** and they were meaningful because:

Today I decide to ***improve*** myself in this way:

To improve, I will be aware of this ***trigger*** happening in the future:

I ***decide*** now that if a similar trigger situation arises in the future, I will do this:

Day #34 Date: ______

Morning Preparation

My long-term ***vision*** is:

This morning I am ***grateful*** for... and it is meaningful because:

Today I ***intend*** to be:

Today I will ***focus*** my attention on these tasks which will help me achieve my vision:

Evening Review

Today I intentionally performed this act of ***kindness*** and I learned:

Today I had these ***successes*** and they were meaningful because:

Today I decide to ***improve*** myself in this way:

To improve, I will be aware of this ***trigger*** happening in the future:

I ***decide*** now that if a similar trigger situation arises in the future, I will do this:

DAY #35 Date: ______

Morning Preparation

My long-term ***vision*** is:

This morning I am ***grateful*** for... and it is meaningful because:

Today I ***intend*** to be:

Today I will ***focus*** my attention on these tasks which will help me achieve my vision:

Evening Review

Today I intentionally performed this act of ***kindness*** and I learned:

Today I had these ***successes*** and they were meaningful because:

Today I decide to ***improve*** myself in this way:

To improve, I will be aware of this ***trigger*** happening in the future:

I ***decide*** now that if a similar trigger situation arises in the future, I will do this:

DAY #36 Date: ______

Morning Preparation

My long-term ***vision*** is:

This morning I am ***grateful*** for... and it is meaningful because:

Today I ***intend*** to be:

Today I will ***focus*** my attention on these tasks which will help me achieve my vision:

Evening Review

Today I intentionally performed this act of ***kindness*** and I learned:

Today I had these ***successes*** and they were meaningful because:

Today I decide to ***improve*** myself in this way:

To improve, I will be aware of this ***trigger*** happening in the future:

I ***decide*** now that if a similar trigger situation arises in the future, I will do this:

DAY #37 Date: ______

Morning Preparation

My long-term ***vision*** is:

This morning I am ***grateful*** for... and it is meaningful because:

Today I ***intend*** to be:

Today I will ***focus*** my attention on these tasks which will help me achieve my vision:

Evening Review

Today I intentionally performed this act of ***kindness*** and I learned:

Today I had these ***successes*** and they were meaningful because:

Today I decide to ***improve*** myself in this way:

To improve, I will be aware of this ***trigger*** happening in the future:

I ***decide*** now that if a similar trigger situation arises in the future, I will do this:

DAY #38 Date: ______

Morning Preparation

My long-term ***vision*** is:

This morning I am ***grateful*** for... and it is meaningful because:

Today I ***intend*** to be:

Today I will ***focus*** my attention on these tasks which will help me achieve my vision:

Evening Review

Today I intentionally performed this act of ***kindness*** and I learned:

Today I had these ***successes*** and they were meaningful because:

Today I decide to ***improve*** myself in this way:

To improve, I will be aware of this ***trigger*** happening in the future:

I ***decide*** now that if a similar trigger situation arises in the future, I will do this:

Day #39 Date: ______

Morning Preparation

My long-term ***vision*** is:

This morning I am ***grateful*** for... and it is meaningful because:

Today I ***intend*** to be:

Today I will ***focus*** my attention on these tasks which will help me achieve my vision:

Evening Review

Today I intentionally performed this act of ***kindness*** and I learned:

Today I had these ***successes*** and they were meaningful because:

Today I decide to ***improve*** myself in this way:

To improve, I will be aware of this ***trigger*** happening in the future:

I ***decide*** now that if a similar trigger situation arises in the future, I will do this:

Day #40 Date: ______

Morning Preparation

My long-term ***vision*** is:

This morning I am ***grateful*** for... and it is meaningful because:

Today I ***intend*** to be:

Today I will ***focus*** my attention on these tasks which will help me achieve my vision:

Evening Review

Today I intentionally performed this act of ***kindness*** and I learned:

Today I had these ***successes*** and they were meaningful because:

Today I decide to ***improve*** myself in this way:

To improve, I will be aware of this ***trigger*** happening in the future:

I ***decide*** now that if a similar trigger situation arises in the future, I will do this:

Day #41 Date: ______

Morning Preparation

My long-term ***vision*** is:

This morning I am ***grateful*** for... and it is meaningful because:

Today I ***intend*** to be:

Today I will ***focus*** my attention on these tasks which will help me achieve my vision:

Evening Review

Today I intentionally performed this act of ***kindness*** and I learned:

Today I had these ***successes*** and they were meaningful because:

Today I decide to ***improve*** myself in this way:

To improve, I will be aware of this ***trigger*** happening in the future:

I ***decide*** now that if a similar trigger situation arises in the future, I will do this:

DAY #42 Date: ______

Morning Preparation

My long-term ***vision*** is:

This morning I am ***grateful*** for... and it is meaningful because:

Today I ***intend*** to be:

Today I will ***focus*** my attention on these tasks which will help me achieve my vision:

Evening Review

Today I intentionally performed this act of ***kindness*** and I learned:

Today I had these ***successes*** and they were meaningful because:

Today I decide to ***improve*** myself in this way:

To improve, I will be aware of this ***trigger*** happening in the future:

I ***decide*** now that if a similar trigger situation arises in the future, I will do this:

DAY #43 Date: ______

Morning Preparation

My long-term ***vision*** is:

This morning I am ***grateful*** for... and it is meaningful because:

Today I ***intend*** to be:

Today I will ***focus*** my attention on these tasks which will help me achieve my vision:

Evening Review

Today I intentionally performed this act of ***kindness*** and I learned:

Today I had these ***successes*** and they were meaningful because:

Today I decide to ***improve*** myself in this way:

To improve, I will be aware of this ***trigger*** happening in the future:

I ***decide*** now that if a similar trigger situation arises in the future, I will do this:

DAY #44 Date: ______

Morning Preparation

My long-term ***vision*** is:

This morning I am ***grateful*** for... and it is meaningful because:

Today I ***intend*** to be:

Today I will ***focus*** my attention on these tasks which will help me achieve my vision:

Evening Review

Today I intentionally performed this act of ***kindness*** and I learned:

Today I had these ***successes*** and they were meaningful because:

Today I decide to ***improve*** myself in this way:

To improve, I will be aware of this ***trigger*** happening in the future:

I ***decide*** now that if a similar trigger situation arises in the future, I will do this:

DAY #45 Date: ______

Morning Preparation

My long-term ***vision*** is:

This morning I am ***grateful*** for... and it is meaningful because:

Today I ***intend*** to be:

Today I will ***focus*** my attention on these tasks which will help me achieve my vision:

Evening Review

Today I intentionally performed this act of ***kindness*** and I learned:

Today I had these ***successes*** and they were meaningful because:

Today I decide to ***improve*** myself in this way:

To improve, I will be aware of this ***trigger*** happening in the future:

I ***decide*** now that if a similar trigger situation arises in the future, I will do this:

DAY #46 Date: ______

Morning Preparation

My long-term ***vision*** is:

____

____

____

____

This morning I am ***grateful*** for... and it is meaningful because:

____

____

____

____

Today I ***intend*** to be:

____

____

____

____

Today I will ***focus*** my attention on these tasks which will help me achieve my vision:

____

____

____

____

____

Evening Review

Today I intentionally performed this act of ***kindness*** and I learned:

Today I had these ***successes*** and they were meaningful because:

Today I decide to ***improve*** myself in this way:

To improve, I will be aware of this ***trigger*** happening in the future:

I ***decide*** now that if a similar trigger situation arises in the future, I will do this:

DAY #47 Date: ______

Morning Preparation

My long-term ***vision*** is:

This morning I am ***grateful*** for... and it is meaningful because:

Today I ***intend*** to be:

Today I will ***focus*** my attention on these tasks which will help me achieve my vision:

Evening Review

Today I intentionally performed this act of ***kindness*** and I learned:

Today I had these ***successes*** and they were meaningful because:

Today I decide to ***improve*** myself in this way:

To improve, I will be aware of this ***trigger*** happening in the future:

I ***decide*** now that if a similar trigger situation arises in the future, I will do this:

Day #48 Date: ______

Morning Preparation

My long-term ***vision*** is:

This morning I am ***grateful*** for... and it is meaningful because:

Today I ***intend*** to be:

Today I will ***focus*** my attention on these tasks which will help me achieve my vision:

Evening Review

Today I intentionally performed this act of ***kindness*** and I learned:

Today I had these ***successes*** and they were meaningful because:

Today I decide to ***improve*** myself in this way:

To improve, I will be aware of this ***trigger*** happening in the future:

I ***decide*** now that if a similar trigger situation arises in the future, I will do this:

DAY #49 Date: ______

Morning Preparation

My long-term ***vision*** is:

This morning I am ***grateful*** for... and it is meaningful because:

Today I ***intend*** to be:

Today I will ***focus*** my attention on these tasks which will help me achieve my vision:

Evening Review

Today I intentionally performed this act of ***kindness*** and I learned:

Today I had these ***successes*** and they were meaningful because:

Today I decide to ***improve*** myself in this way:

To improve, I will be aware of this ***trigger*** happening in the future:

I ***decide*** now that if a similar trigger situation arises in the future, I will do this:

Day #50 Date: ______

Morning Preparation

My long-term ***vision*** is:

This morning I am ***grateful*** for... and it is meaningful because:

Today I ***intend*** to be:

Today I will ***focus*** my attention on these tasks which will help me achieve my vision:

Evening Review

Today I intentionally performed this act of ***kindness*** and I learned:

Today I had these ***successes*** and they were meaningful because:

Today I decide to ***improve*** myself in this way:

To improve, I will be aware of this ***trigger*** happening in the future:

I ***decide*** now that if a similar trigger situation arises in the future, I will do this:

Day #51 Date: ______

Morning Preparation

My long-term ***vision*** is:

This morning I am ***grateful*** for... and it is meaningful because:

Today I ***intend*** to be:

Today I will ***focus*** my attention on these tasks which will help me achieve my vision:

Evening Review

Today I intentionally performed this act of ***kindness*** and I learned:

Today I had these ***successes*** and they were meaningful because:

Today I decide to ***improve*** myself in this way:

To improve, I will be aware of this ***trigger*** happening in the future:

I ***decide*** now that if a similar trigger situation arises in the future, I will do this:

Day #52 Date: ______

Morning Preparation

My long-term ***vision*** is:

This morning I am ***grateful*** for... and it is meaningful because:

Today I ***intend*** to be:

Today I will ***focus*** my attention on these tasks which will help me achieve my vision:

Evening Review

Today I intentionally performed this act of ***kindness*** and I learned:

Today I had these ***successes*** and they were meaningful because:

Today I decide to ***improve*** myself in this way:

To improve, I will be aware of this ***trigger*** happening in the future:

I ***decide*** now that if a similar trigger situation arises in the future, I will do this:

DAY #53 Date: ______

Morning Preparation

My long-term ***vision*** is:

This morning I am ***grateful*** for... and it is meaningful because:

Today I ***intend*** to be:

Today I will ***focus*** my attention on these tasks which will help me achieve my vision:

Evening Review

Today I intentionally performed this act of ***kindness*** and I learned:

Today I had these ***successes*** and they were meaningful because:

Today I decide to ***improve*** myself in this way:

To improve, I will be aware of this ***trigger*** happening in the future:

I ***decide*** now that if a similar trigger situation arises in the future, I will do this:

Day #54 Date: ______

Morning Preparation

My long-term ***vision*** is:

This morning I am ***grateful*** for... and it is meaningful because:

Today I ***intend*** to be:

Today I will ***focus*** my attention on these tasks which will help me achieve my vision:

Evening Review

Today I intentionally performed this act of ***kindness*** and I learned:

Today I had these ***successes*** and they were meaningful because:

Today I decide to ***improve*** myself in this way:

To improve, I will be aware of this ***trigger*** happening in the future:

I ***decide*** now that if a similar trigger situation arises in the future, I will do this:

Day #55 Date: ______

Morning Preparation

My long-term ***vision*** is:

This morning I am ***grateful*** for... and it is meaningful because:

Today I ***intend*** to be:

Today I will ***focus*** my attention on these tasks which will help me achieve my vision:

Evening Review

Today I intentionally performed this act of ***kindness*** and I learned:

Today I had these ***successes*** and they were meaningful because:

Today I decide to ***improve*** myself in this way:

To improve, I will be aware of this ***trigger*** happening in the future:

I ***decide*** now that if a similar trigger situation arises in the future, I will do this:

DAY #56 Date: ______

Morning Preparation

My long-term ***vision*** is:

This morning I am ***grateful*** for... and it is meaningful because:

Today I ***intend*** to be:

Today I will ***focus*** my attention on these tasks which will help me achieve my vision:

Evening Review

Today I intentionally performed this act of ***kindness*** and I learned:

Today I had these ***successes*** and they were meaningful because:

Today I decide to ***improve*** myself in this way:

To improve, I will be aware of this ***trigger*** happening in the future:

I ***decide*** now that if a similar trigger situation arises in the future, I will do this:

Day #57 Date: ______

Morning Preparation

My long-term ***vision*** is:

This morning I am ***grateful*** for... and it is meaningful because:

Today I ***intend*** to be:

Today I will ***focus*** my attention on these tasks which will help me achieve my vision:

Evening Review

Today I intentionally performed this act of ***kindness*** and I learned:

Today I had these ***successes*** and they were meaningful because:

Today I decide to ***improve*** myself in this way:

To improve, I will be aware of this ***trigger*** happening in the future:

I ***decide*** now that if a similar trigger situation arises in the future, I will do this:

DAY #58 Date: ______

Morning Preparation

My long-term ***vision*** is:

This morning I am ***grateful*** for... and it is meaningful because:

Today I ***intend*** to be:

Today I will ***focus*** my attention on these tasks which will help me achieve my vision:

Evening Review

Today I intentionally performed this act of ***kindness*** and I learned:

Today I had these ***successes*** and they were meaningful because:

Today I decide to ***improve*** myself in this way:

To improve, I will be aware of this ***trigger*** happening in the future:

I ***decide*** now that if a similar trigger situation arises in the future, I will do this:

DAY #59 Date: ______

Morning Preparation

My long-term ***vision*** is:

This morning I am ***grateful*** for... and it is meaningful because:

Today I ***intend*** to be:

Today I will ***focus*** my attention on these tasks which will help me achieve my vision:

Evening Review

Today I intentionally performed this act of ***kindness*** and I learned:

Today I had these ***successes*** and they were meaningful because:

Today I decide to ***improve*** myself in this way:

To improve, I will be aware of this ***trigger*** happening in the future:

I ***decide*** now that if a similar trigger situation arises in the future, I will do this:

DAY #60 Date: ______

Morning Preparation

My long-term ***vision*** is:

This morning I am ***grateful*** for... and it is meaningful because:

Today I ***intend*** to be:

Today I will ***focus*** my attention on these tasks which will help me achieve my vision:

Evening Review

Today I intentionally performed this act of ***kindness*** and I learned:

Today I had these ***successes*** and they were meaningful because:

Today I decide to ***improve*** myself in this way:

To improve, I will be aware of this ***trigger*** happening in the future:

I ***decide*** now that if a similar trigger situation arises in the future, I will do this:

DAY #61 Date: ______

Morning Preparation

My long-term ***vision*** is:

This morning I am ***grateful*** for... and it is meaningful because:

Today I ***intend*** to be:

Today I will ***focus*** my attention on these tasks which will help me achieve my vision:

Evening Review

Today I intentionally performed this act of ***kindness*** and I learned:

Today I had these ***successes*** and they were meaningful because:

Today I decide to ***improve*** myself in this way:

To improve, I will be aware of this ***trigger*** happening in the future:

I ***decide*** now that if a similar trigger situation arises in the future, I will do this:

DAY #62 Date: ______

Morning Preparation

My long-term ***vision*** is:

This morning I am ***grateful*** for... and it is meaningful because:

Today I ***intend*** to be:

Today I will ***focus*** my attention on these tasks which will help me achieve my vision:

Evening Review

Today I intentionally performed this act of ***kindness*** and I learned:

Today I had these ***successes*** and they were meaningful because:

Today I decide to ***improve*** myself in this way:

To improve, I will be aware of this ***trigger*** happening in the future:

I ***decide*** now that if a similar trigger situation arises in the future, I will do this:

Day #63 Date: ______

Morning Preparation

My long-term ***vision*** is:

This morning I am ***grateful*** for... and it is meaningful because:

Today I ***intend*** to be:

Today I will ***focus*** my attention on these tasks which will help me achieve my vision:

Evening Review

Today I intentionally performed this act of ***kindness*** and I learned:

Today I had these ***successes*** and they were meaningful because:

Today I decide to ***improve*** myself in this way:

To improve, I will be aware of this ***trigger*** happening in the future:

I ***decide*** now that if a similar trigger situation arises in the future, I will do this:

Day #64 Date: ______

Morning Preparation

My long-term ***vision*** is:

This morning I am ***grateful*** for... and it is meaningful because:

Today I ***intend*** to be:

Today I will ***focus*** my attention on these tasks which will help me achieve my vision:

Evening Review

Today I intentionally performed this act of ***kindness*** and I learned:

Today I had these ***successes*** and they were meaningful because:

Today I decide to ***improve*** myself in this way:

To improve, I will be aware of this ***trigger*** happening in the future:

I ***decide*** now that if a similar trigger situation arises in the future, I will do this:

Day #65 Date: ______

Morning Preparation

My long-term ***vision*** is:

This morning I am ***grateful*** for... and it is meaningful because:

Today I ***intend*** to be:

Today I will ***focus*** my attention on these tasks which will help me achieve my vision:

Evening Review

Today I intentionally performed this act of ***kindness*** and I learned:

Today I had these ***successes*** and they were meaningful because:

Today I decide to ***improve*** myself in this way:

To improve, I will be aware of this ***trigger*** happening in the future:

I ***decide*** now that if a similar trigger situation arises in the future, I will do this:

DAY #66 Date: ______

Morning Preparation

My long-term ***vision*** is:

This morning I am ***grateful*** for... and it is meaningful because:

Today I ***intend*** to be:

Today I will ***focus*** my attention on these tasks which will help me achieve my vision:

Evening Review

Today I intentionally performed this act of ***kindness*** and I learned:

Today I had these ***successes*** and they were meaningful because:

Today I decide to ***improve*** myself in this way:

To improve, I will be aware of this ***trigger*** happening in the future:

I ***decide*** now that if a similar trigger situation arises in the future, I will do this:

DAY #67 Date: ______

Morning Preparation

My long-term ***vision*** is:

This morning I am ***grateful*** for... and it is meaningful because:

Today I ***intend*** to be:

Today I will ***focus*** my attention on these tasks which will help me achieve my vision:

Evening Review

Today I intentionally performed this act of ***kindness*** and I learned:

Today I had these ***successes*** and they were meaningful because:

Today I decide to ***improve*** myself in this way:

To improve, I will be aware of this ***trigger*** happening in the future:

I ***decide*** now that if a similar trigger situation arises in the future, I will do this:

DAY #68 Date: ______

Morning Preparation

My long-term ***vision*** is:

This morning I am ***grateful*** for... and it is meaningful because:

Today I ***intend*** to be:

Today I will ***focus*** my attention on these tasks which will help me achieve my vision:

Evening Review

Today I intentionally performed this act of ***kindness*** and I learned:

Today I had these ***successes*** and they were meaningful because:

Today I decide to ***improve*** myself in this way:

To improve, I will be aware of this ***trigger*** happening in the future:

I ***decide*** now that if a similar trigger situation arises in the future, I will do this:

Day #69 Date: ______

Morning Preparation

My long-term ***vision*** is:

This morning I am ***grateful*** for... and it is meaningful because:

Today I ***intend*** to be:

Today I will ***focus*** my attention on these tasks which will help me achieve my vision:

Evening Review

Today I intentionally performed this act of ***kindness*** and I learned:

Today I had these ***successes*** and they were meaningful because:

Today I decide to ***improve*** myself in this way:

To improve, I will be aware of this ***trigger*** happening in the future:

I ***decide*** now that if a similar trigger situation arises in the future, I will do this:

Day #70 Date: ______

Morning Preparation

My long-term ***vision*** is:

This morning I am ***grateful*** for... and it is meaningful because:

Today I ***intend*** to be:

Today I will ***focus*** my attention on these tasks which will help me achieve my vision:

Evening Review

Today I intentionally performed this act of ***kindness*** and I learned:

Today I had these ***successes*** and they were meaningful because:

Today I decide to ***improve*** myself in this way:

To improve, I will be aware of this ***trigger*** happening in the future:

I ***decide*** now that if a similar trigger situation arises in the future, I will do this:

DAY #71 Date: ______

Morning Preparation

My long-term ***vision*** is:

This morning I am ***grateful*** for... and it is meaningful because:

Today I ***intend*** to be:

Today I will ***focus*** my attention on these tasks which will help me achieve my vision:

Evening Review

Today I intentionally performed this act of ***kindness*** and I learned:

Today I had these ***successes*** and they were meaningful because:

Today I decide to ***improve*** myself in this way:

To improve, I will be aware of this ***trigger*** happening in the future:

I ***decide*** now that if a similar trigger situation arises in the future, I will do this:

Day #72 Date: ______

Morning Preparation

My long-term ***vision*** is:

This morning I am ***grateful*** for... and it is meaningful because:

Today I ***intend*** to be:

Today I will ***focus*** my attention on these tasks which will help me achieve my vision:

Evening Review

Today I intentionally performed this act of ***kindness*** and I learned:

Today I had these ***successes*** and they were meaningful because:

Today I decide to ***improve*** myself in this way:

To improve, I will be aware of this ***trigger*** happening in the future:

I ***decide*** now that if a similar trigger situation arises in the future, I will do this:

DAY #73 Date: ______

Morning Preparation

My long-term ***vision*** is:

This morning I am ***grateful*** for... and it is meaningful because:

Today I ***intend*** to be:

Today I will ***focus*** my attention on these tasks which will help me achieve my vision:

Evening Review

Today I intentionally performed this act of ***kindness*** and I learned:

Today I had these ***successes*** and they were meaningful because:

Today I decide to ***improve*** myself in this way:

To improve, I will be aware of this ***trigger*** happening in the future:

I ***decide*** now that if a similar trigger situation arises in the future, I will do this:

DAY #74 Date: ______

Morning Preparation

My long-term ***vision*** is:

This morning I am ***grateful*** for... and it is meaningful because:

Today I ***intend*** to be:

Today I will ***focus*** my attention on these tasks which will help me achieve my vision:

Evening Review

Today I intentionally performed this act of ***kindness*** and I learned:

Today I had these ***successes*** and they were meaningful because:

Today I decide to ***improve*** myself in this way:

To improve, I will be aware of this ***trigger*** happening in the future:

I ***decide*** now that if a similar trigger situation arises in the future, I will do this:

Day #75 Date: ______

Morning Preparation

My long-term ***vision*** is:

This morning I am ***grateful*** for... and it is meaningful because:

Today I ***intend*** to be:

Today I will ***focus*** my attention on these tasks which will help me achieve my vision:

Evening Review

Today I intentionally performed this act of ***kindness*** and I learned:

Today I had these ***successes*** and they were meaningful because:

Today I decide to ***improve*** myself in this way:

To improve, I will be aware of this ***trigger*** happening in the future:

I ***decide*** now that if a similar trigger situation arises in the future, I will do this:

DAY #76 Date: ______

Morning Preparation

My long-term ***vision*** is:

This morning I am ***grateful*** for... and it is meaningful because:

Today I ***intend*** to be:

Today I will ***focus*** my attention on these tasks which will help me achieve my vision:

Evening Review

Today I intentionally performed this act of ***kindness*** and I learned:

Today I had these ***successes*** and they were meaningful because:

Today I decide to ***improve*** myself in this way:

To improve, I will be aware of this ***trigger*** happening in the future:

I ***decide*** now that if a similar trigger situation arises in the future, I will do this:

Day #77 Date: ______

Morning Preparation

My long-term ***vision*** is:

This morning I am ***grateful*** for... and it is meaningful because:

Today I ***intend*** to be:

Today I will ***focus*** my attention on these tasks which will help me achieve my vision:

Evening Review

Today I intentionally performed this act of ***kindness*** and I learned:

Today I had these ***successes*** and they were meaningful because:

Today I decide to ***improve*** myself in this way:

To improve, I will be aware of this ***trigger*** happening in the future:

I ***decide*** now that if a similar trigger situation arises in the future, I will do this:

Day #78 Date: ______

Morning Preparation

My long-term ***vision*** is:

This morning I am ***grateful*** for... and it is meaningful because:

Today I ***intend*** to be:

Today I will ***focus*** my attention on these tasks which will help me achieve my vision:

Evening Review

Today I intentionally performed this act of ***kindness*** and I learned:

Today I had these ***successes*** and they were meaningful because:

Today I decide to ***improve*** myself in this way:

To improve, I will be aware of this ***trigger*** happening in the future:

I ***decide*** now that if a similar trigger situation arises in the future, I will do this:

DAY #79 Date: ______

Morning Preparation

My long-term ***vision*** is:

This morning I am ***grateful*** for... and it is meaningful because:

Today I ***intend*** to be:

Today I will ***focus*** my attention on these tasks which will help me achieve my vision:

Evening Review

Today I intentionally performed this act of ***kindness*** and I learned:

Today I had these ***successes*** and they were meaningful because:

Today I decide to ***improve*** myself in this way:

To improve, I will be aware of this ***trigger*** happening in the future:

I ***decide*** now that if a similar trigger situation arises in the future, I will do this:

DAY #80 Date: ______

Morning Preparation

My long-term ***vision*** is:

This morning I am ***grateful*** for... and it is meaningful because:

Today I ***intend*** to be:

Today I will ***focus*** my attention on these tasks which will help me achieve my vision:

Evening Review

Today I intentionally performed this act of ***kindness*** and I learned:

Today I had these ***successes*** and they were meaningful because:

Today I decide to ***improve*** myself in this way:

To improve, I will be aware of this ***trigger*** happening in the future:

I ***decide*** now that if a similar trigger situation arises in the future, I will do this:

DAY #81 Date: ______

Morning Preparation

My long-term ***vision*** is:

This morning I am ***grateful*** for... and it is meaningful because:

Today I ***intend*** to be:

Today I will ***focus*** my attention on these tasks which will help me achieve my vision:

Evening Review

Today I intentionally performed this act of ***kindness*** and I learned:

Today I had these ***successes*** and they were meaningful because:

Today I decide to ***improve*** myself in this way:

To improve, I will be aware of this ***trigger*** happening in the future:

I ***decide*** now that if a similar trigger situation arises in the future, I will do this:

DAY #82 Date: ______

Morning Preparation

My long-term ***vision*** is:

This morning I am ***grateful*** for... and it is meaningful because:

Today I ***intend*** to be:

Today I will ***focus*** my attention on these tasks which will help me achieve my vision:

Evening Review

Today I intentionally performed this act of ***kindness*** and I learned:

Today I had these ***successes*** and they were meaningful because:

Today I decide to ***improve*** myself in this way:

To improve, I will be aware of this ***trigger*** happening in the future:

I ***decide*** now that if a similar trigger situation arises in the future, I will do this:

DAY #83 Date: ______

Morning Preparation

My long-term ***vision*** is:

This morning I am ***grateful*** for... and it is meaningful because:

Today I ***intend*** to be:

Today I will ***focus*** my attention on these tasks which will help me achieve my vision:

Evening Review

Today I intentionally performed this act of ***kindness*** and I learned:

Today I had these ***successes*** and they were meaningful because:

Today I decide to ***improve*** myself in this way:

To improve, I will be aware of this ***trigger*** happening in the future:

I ***decide*** now that if a similar trigger situation arises in the future, I will do this:

DAY #84 Date: ______

Morning Preparation

My long-term ***vision*** is:

This morning I am ***grateful*** for... and it is meaningful because:

Today I ***intend*** to be:

Today I will ***focus*** my attention on these tasks which will help me achieve my vision:

Evening Review

Today I intentionally performed this act of ***kindness*** and I learned:

Today I had these ***successes*** and they were meaningful because:

Today I decide to ***improve*** myself in this way:

To improve, I will be aware of this ***trigger*** happening in the future:

I ***decide*** now that if a similar trigger situation arises in the future, I will do this:

DAY #85 Date: ______

Morning Preparation

My long-term ***vision*** is:

This morning I am ***grateful*** for... and it is meaningful because:

Today I ***intend*** to be:

Today I will ***focus*** my attention on these tasks which will help me achieve my vision:

Evening Review

Today I intentionally performed this act of ***kindness*** and I learned:

Today I had these ***successes*** and they were meaningful because:

Today I decide to ***improve*** myself in this way:

To improve, I will be aware of this ***trigger*** happening in the future:

I ***decide*** now that if a similar trigger situation arises in the future, I will do this:

DAY #86 Date: ______

Morning Preparation

My long-term ***vision*** is:

This morning I am ***grateful*** for... and it is meaningful because:

Today I ***intend*** to be:

Today I will ***focus*** my attention on these tasks which will help me achieve my vision:

Evening Review

Today I intentionally performed this act of ***kindness*** and I learned:

Today I had these ***successes*** and they were meaningful because:

Today I decide to ***improve*** myself in this way:

To improve, I will be aware of this ***trigger*** happening in the future:

I ***decide*** now that if a similar trigger situation arises in the future, I will do this:

Day #87 Date: ______

Morning Preparation

My long-term ***vision*** is:

This morning I am ***grateful*** for... and it is meaningful because:

Today I ***intend*** to be:

Today I will ***focus*** my attention on these tasks which will help me achieve my vision:

Evening Review

Today I intentionally performed this act of ***kindness*** and I learned:

Today I had these ***successes*** and they were meaningful because:

Today I decide to ***improve*** myself in this way:

To improve, I will be aware of this ***trigger*** happening in the future:

I ***decide*** now that if a similar trigger situation arises in the future, I will do this:

Day #88 Date: ______

Morning Preparation

My long-term ***vision*** is:

This morning I am ***grateful*** for... and it is meaningful because:

Today I ***intend*** to be:

Today I will ***focus*** my attention on these tasks which will help me achieve my vision:

Evening Review

Today I intentionally performed this act of ***kindness*** and I learned:

Today I had these ***successes*** and they were meaningful because:

Today I decide to ***improve*** myself in this way:

To improve, I will be aware of this ***trigger*** happening in the future:

I ***decide*** now that if a similar trigger situation arises in the future, I will do this:

Day #89 Date: ______

Morning Preparation

My long-term ***vision*** is:

This morning I am ***grateful*** for... and it is meaningful because:

Today I ***intend*** to be:

Today I will ***focus*** my attention on these tasks which will help me achieve my vision:

Evening Review

Today I intentionally performed this act of ***kindness*** and I learned:

Today I had these ***successes*** and they were meaningful because:

Today I decide to ***improve*** myself in this way:

To improve, I will be aware of this ***trigger*** happening in the future:

I ***decide*** now that if a similar trigger situation arises in the future, I will do this:

DAY #90 Date: ______

Morning Preparation

My long-term ***vision*** is:

This morning I am ***grateful*** for... and it is meaningful because:

Today I ***intend*** to be:

Today I will ***focus*** my attention on these tasks which will help me achieve my vision:

Evening Review

Today I intentionally performed this act of ***kindness*** and I learned:

Today I had these ***successes*** and they were meaningful because:

Today I decide to ***improve*** myself in this way:

To improve, I will be aware of this ***trigger*** happening in the future:

I ***decide*** now that if a similar trigger situation arises in the future, I will do this:

What's Next?

Congratulations on completing your Brave Leadership Mastery Journal!

You can repeat this 90-day process as often as you like.

The main benefit is that you will continually grow your self awareness, your emotional resilience, and your Brave Leadership Mastery skills.

You also have a resource to track your journey and to reflect on the tremendous successes of your past. In fact, one high school student was so impressed with the practice of documenting at least three successes a night that she exclaimed, "Wow! I would have about 100 successes a month and over 1,000 in a year. This is amazing."

Imagine that for yourself.

You can see a grand list of the decisions you made to impact the moments of your life, and you can see how you have altered the trajectory of your life and human history as a result.

For more information about other Brave Leadership Mastery resources and programs, or to order another Brave Leadership Mastery Journal, go to www.TonyBodoh.com/BLM.

About The Author

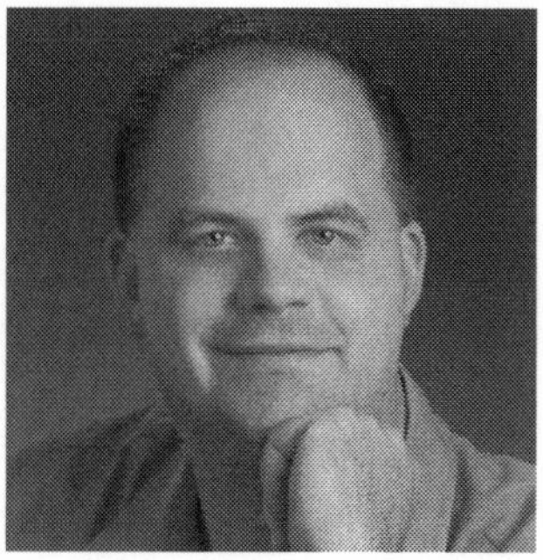

Tony Bodoh is an international speaker, three time best-selling author, consultant & coach to Fortune 1000 executives.

He combines his expertise in human experience & business analytics to help companies create 5-star customer experiences that disrupt their competitors and earn them prestigious awards and rankings from J.D. Power, Temkin Group, ACSI, and TripAdvisor.

In 2018 Tony was named one of the Top 16 Customer Service Movers and Shakers to Follow by the Miller Heiman Group.

Beyond the boardroom, Tony provides highly-acclaimed mental performance training to Olympians, professional athletes, & the U.S. military.

www.TonyBodoh.com

Made in the USA
Coppell, TX
10 January 2024

27497079R00111